THE SUPERCHARGED DIVERTICULITIS DIET COOKBOOK, FOOD LIST, AND MEAL PLAN FOR SENIORS

What to Eat and What to Avoid, Understanding Symptoms, Effective Diagnosis, and Strategies for Prevention and Recovery—All You Need to Live Pain-Free.

Dr. Olivia Karyn Gray

TABLE OF CONTENTS

INTRODUCTION

Welcome to "The Supercharged Diverticulitis Diet Cookbook, Food List, and Meal Plan for Seniors"! If you're holding this book, chances are you or someone you care about is navigating the challenges of living with diverticulitis. You're not alone in this journey, and I want you to know that I understand how overwhelming it can be to balance delicious meals with managing your health.

As we age, our bodies change, and health concerns like diverticulitis can sometimes feel like unexpected roadblocks on the path to enjoying life to the fullest. But fear not! This book is your guide to not just managing but thriving with diverticulitis.

On these pages, you'll find more than just a collection of recipes. You'll discover a comprehensive approach to managing diverticulitis through the power of nutrition. We'll delve into the foods that can soothe your digestive system, boost your energy levels, and tantalize your taste buds—all while keeping your health front and center.

Whether you're a seasoned cook looking for new inspiration in the kitchen or someone who's just starting to explore the world of dietary management for diverticulitis, this book is designed with you in mind. From practical kitchen tips to mouthwatering recipes and easy-to-follow meal plans, we've got everything you need to embark on your journey to better health, one delicious bite at a time.

CHAPTER ONE

UNDERSTANDING DIVERTICULITIS

What is Diverticulitis?

Diverticulitis is a common digestive condition characterized by inflammation or infection of small pouches called diverticula that form along the walls of the colon or large intestine. These pouches, known as diverticula, can develop when weak areas in the colon's muscular wall bulge outward, creating small pockets. While diverticulosis refers to the presence of these pouches without inflammation or infection, diverticulitis occurs when these pouches become inflamed or infected, leading to various symptoms ranging from mild discomfort to severe complications.

Causes and Risk Factors

The exact cause of diverticulitis is not fully understood, but several factors are believed to contribute to its development. One primary factor is thought to be a diet low in fiber, which can result in constipation and increased pressure within the colon, leading to the formation of diverticula. Other risk factors include aging, genetics, obesity, lack of exercise, smoking, and certain medications such as nonsteroidal anti-inflammatory drugs (NSAIDs).

Symptoms and Diagnosis

Symptoms of diverticulitis can vary in severity and may include abdominal pain, particularly in the lower left side, bloating, fever, nausea, vomiting, changes in bowel habits, such as diarrhea or constipation, and rectal bleeding. However, not all individuals with diverticulitis will experience symptoms, and some may only have mild discomfort.

Diagnosing diverticulitis typically involves a combination of medical history evaluation, physical examination, and diagnostic tests. During the physical exam, your healthcare provider may press on your abdomen to check for tenderness or signs of inflammation. Blood tests may also be ordered to check for signs of infection, such as an elevated white blood cell count. Imaging tests, such as a CT scan or abdominal ultrasound, may be used to confirm the diagnosis and assess the severity of the condition.

Treatment Options

Treatment for diverticulitis depends on the severity of symptoms and the presence of complications. In mild cases, treatment may involve conservative measures such as dietary modifications, rest, and over-the-counter pain relievers to alleviate discomfort. Increasing fiber intake and staying hydrated can help soften stools and promote regular bowel movements, reducing the risk of further inflammation or infection.

In more severe cases or when complications arise, such as abscess formation or bowel obstruction, medical intervention may be necessary. Antibiotics are often prescribed to treat infection, while pain medications may be given to manage discomfort. In some cases, a liquid or low-fiber diet may be recommended to give the colon time to heal. In severe or recurrent cases, hospitalization may be required for intravenous antibiotics and supportive care.

In rare instances where complications persist or recur despite conservative treatment, surgical intervention may be necessary. Surgery may involve removing the affected portion of the colon (resection) or creating a temporary or permanent colostomy to divert stool away from the affected area. Surgical options vary depending on the individual's condition and overall health.

CHAPTER TWO
IMPORTANCE OF DIET IN MANAGING DIVERTICULITIS

Role of Diet in Prevention and Management

Diet plays a crucial role in both the prevention and management of diverticulitis. Making healthy dietary choices can help prevent the formation of diverticula and reduce the risk of inflammation or infection. Additionally, following a specific diet can help manage symptoms and alleviate discomfort associated with diverticulitis flare-ups. Let's explore the role of diet in more detail and how you can optimize your eating habits to promote digestive health.

Prevention

Preventing diverticulitis starts with maintaining a diet rich in fiber. Fiber plays a key role in promoting regular bowel movements and preventing constipation, which can contribute to the development of diverticula. A high-fiber diet softens stools and makes them easier to pass, reducing pressure on the colon walls and decreasing the risk of diverticula formation.

Foods high in fiber include fruits, vegetables, whole grains, legumes, nuts, and seeds. Aim to incorporate a variety of these fiber-rich foods into your daily meals and snacks to meet your dietary fiber needs. Gradually increasing fiber intake over time can help prevent bloating and gas commonly associated with sudden changes in dietary fiber.

Management

For individuals already diagnosed with diverticulitis, dietary management plays a crucial role in managing symptoms and preventing flare-ups. While recommendations may vary depending on individual tolerance and preferences, certain dietary guidelines can help alleviate discomfort and promote healing.

Foods to Avoid

Certain foods may exacerbate symptoms or trigger diverticulitis flare-ups and should be avoided or limited in your diet.

These include:

1. **Highly Processed Foods:** Processed foods high in refined sugars, unhealthy fats, and artificial additives can irritate the digestive system and worsen symptoms. Limit consumption of packaged snacks, sugary desserts, and fast food.

2. **Red Meat:** Red meat, particularly fatty cuts, can be difficult to digest and may increase inflammation in the colon. Opt for lean protein sources such as poultry, fish, tofu, and legumes instead.

3. **Dairy Products:** Some individuals with diverticulitis may experience sensitivity to dairy products, especially if lactose

intolerant. Limit consumption of milk, cheese, and yogurt, or opt for lactose-free alternatives.

4. **Spicy Foods:** Spicy foods can irritate the digestive tract and exacerbate symptoms such as abdominal pain and bloating. Avoid or limit the consumption of spicy dishes and condiments.

5. **Seeds and Nuts:** While there is limited scientific evidence linking seeds and nuts to diverticulitis flare-ups, some healthcare providers may recommend avoiding them during acute episodes to reduce the risk of irritation. However, this recommendation may vary among individuals, so it's essential to consult with your healthcare provider for personalized dietary advice.

Foods to Include

On the other hand, certain foods can help soothe the digestive system, reduce inflammation, and promote healing.

Incorporate the following foods into your diet to support digestive health:

1. **High-Fiber Foods:** As mentioned earlier, fiber-rich foods are essential for preventing constipation and promoting regular bowel movements. Include plenty of fruits, vegetables, whole grains, legumes, nuts, and seeds in your meals and snacks.

2. **Probiotic-Rich Foods:** Probiotics are beneficial bacteria that promote a healthy balance of gut flora and support digestive function. Include probiotic-rich foods such as yogurt, kefir, sauerkraut, kimchi, and kombucha in your diet to support gut health.

3. **Omega-3 Fatty Acids:** Omega-3 fatty acids have anti-inflammatory properties and may help reduce inflammation in the digestive tract. Include fatty fish such as salmon, mackerel, and sardines, as well as flaxseeds, chia seeds, and walnuts in your diet to increase your omega-3 intake.

4. **Herbs and Spices:** Certain herbs and spices have anti-inflammatory and digestive benefits and can be incorporated into your cooking to enhance flavor and promote digestive health. Experiment with herbs such as ginger, turmeric, peppermint, and fennel to soothe the digestive system and alleviate symptoms.

5. **Healthy Fats:** Opt for healthy fats such as olive oil, avocado, and nuts, which provide essential nutrients and support overall health without exacerbating inflammation.

CHAPTER THREE

KITCHEN ESSENTIALS AND COOKING

Essential Tools and Equipment

When it comes to cooking nutritious and delicious meals, having the right tools and equipment can make all the difference. Whether you're a seasoned chef or just starting in the kitchen, having a well-stocked kitchen can streamline meal preparation and make cooking more enjoyable.

Let's explore some essential tools and equipment every kitchen should have:

1. **Chef's Knife:** A high-quality chef's knife is arguably the most important tool in any kitchen. Look for a knife with a sharp, sturdy blade and a comfortable handle that fits your hand well. A good chef's knife can make chopping, slicing, and dicing ingredients a breeze, saving you time and effort in the kitchen.

2. **Cutting Board:** A durable cutting board is essential for safely chopping and preparing ingredients. Choose a cutting board made of wood, plastic, or bamboo that is large enough to accommodate your food preparation needs. It's also a good idea to have multiple cutting boards on hand to prevent

cross-contamination between raw meats, poultry, and vegetables.

3. **Cookware Set:** Invest in a high-quality cookware set that includes a variety of pots and pans in different sizes. Look for pots and pans made of stainless steel, nonstick, or cast iron, which are versatile and durable. Having a range of cookware options allows you to cook a wide variety of dishes with ease.

4. **Mixing Bowls:** A set of mixing bowls in various sizes is essential for mixing ingredients, marinating meats, and storing leftovers. Choose bowls made of stainless steel, glass, or plastic that are sturdy and easy to clean. Having a few nesting mixing bowls can help save storage space in your kitchen.

5. **Measuring Cups and Spoons:** Accurate measuring is crucial for achieving consistent results in cooking and baking. Invest in a set of measuring cups and spoons made of durable materials such as stainless steel or plastic. Look for cups and spoons with both standard and metric measurements for versatility.

6. **Kitchen Scale:** While measuring cups and spoons are essential for dry ingredients, a kitchen scale is invaluable for measuring ingredients by weight. A digital kitchen scale allows for precise measurements, especially when it comes to ingredients like flour, sugar, and spices.

7. **Blender or Food Processor:** A blender or food processor is a versatile tool that can be used for everything from making smoothies and soups to chopping vegetables and grinding nuts. Choose a blender or food processor with multiple speed settings and sharp blades for optimal performance.

8. **Baking Sheets and Pans:** If you enjoy baking, having a selection of baking sheets and pans is essential. Look for baking sheets made of heavy-duty aluminum or stainless steel for even heat distribution. Invest in cake pans, muffin tins, and loaf pans for baking a variety of sweet and savory treats.

9. **Kitchen Utensils:** Don't forget about essential kitchen utensils like spatulas, wooden spoons, tongs, and ladles. These tools are indispensable for stirring, flipping, and serving food. Choose utensils made of heat-resistant materials that won't scratch your cookware.

10. **Storage Containers:** Having a variety of storage containers on hand is essential for storing leftovers and meal prepping. Look for containers that are microwave and dishwasher-safe, and consider investing in a set with interchangeable lids for easy storage.

Cooking Methods for Healthy Eating

Now that you have the right tools and equipment in your kitchen.

Let's explore some cooking methods for preparing healthy and nutritious meals:

1. **Grilling:** Grilling is a healthy cooking method that allows you to cook meats, poultry, fish, and vegetables without added fats or oils. Grilling imparts a smoky flavor to food while retaining nutrients and moisture. Use a grill pan or outdoor grill to cook foods quickly and evenly.

2. **Roasting:** Roasting involves cooking food in the oven at high heat, usually around 400-450°F (200-230°C). Roasting is a great way to caramelize vegetables, meats, and poultry, enhancing their natural flavors. Use a rimmed baking sheet or roasting pan to catch any drippings and prevent messes in the oven.

3. **Steaming:** Steaming is a gentle cooking method that preserves the natural flavor, color, and nutrients of the food. Steaming involves cooking food over boiling water in a covered pot or steamer basket. Use a steamer basket or bamboo steamer to steam vegetables, seafood, and dumplings to perfection.

4. **Sauteing:** Sauteing involves cooking food quickly in a small amount of oil or fat over medium-high heat. Sauteing is a great way to cook vegetables, meats, and seafood while

preserving their texture and flavor. Use a nonstick skillet or sauté pan to prevent sticking and ensure even cooking.

5. **Stir-Frying:** Stir-frying is a Chinese cooking technique that involves cooking food quickly in a small amount of oil over high heat. Stir-frying allows you to cook vegetables, meats, and tofu while retaining their crispness and nutrients. Use a wok or large skillet with sloped sides for easy stirring and tossing.

6. **Braising:** Braising is a cooking method that involves searing food in a small amount of fat, and then simmering it in liquid until tender. Braising is ideal for tougher cuts of meat and root vegetables, as it helps break down connective tissue and infuse flavor. Use a Dutch oven or heavy-bottomed pot for braising dishes.

7. **Poaching:** Poaching involves cooking food gently in simmering liquid, such as water, broth, or wine. Poaching is a healthy cooking method that helps retain moisture and flavor without added fats or oils. Use a shallow pan or skillet to poach eggs, fish, chicken, or fruit.

8. **Broiling:** Broiling is a cooking method that involves cooking food under high heat, usually in the oven's top rack. Broiling is similar to grilling but uses direct heat from above instead of below. Use a broiler pan or baking sheet lined with foil to broil meats, poultry, fish, and vegetables until browned and tender.

CHAPTER FOUR

SUPERCHARGED DIVERTICULITIS DIET FOOD LIST

Whole Grains and Cereals

Food Name	Portion Size	Calories (kcal)	Carbohydrates (g)	Fiber (g)	Protein (g)	Fat (g)
Amaranth	1/2 cup	134	24	3	4	2
Barley	1/2 cup	97	21	3	3.5	0.5
Brown Rice	1/2 cup	108	22.5	1.8	2.3	0.9
Brown Rice Cakes	2 cakes	70	14	1	2	0.5
Buckwheat	1/2 cup	154	33	4.5	5	1
Buckwheat Pancakes	2 pancakes	220	43	4	7	3
Bulgur	1/2 cup	76	17	4	3	0.4

Farro	1/2 cup	100	20	3	3.5	0.5
Freekeh	1/2 cup	160	32	4	8	1
Kamut	1/2 cup	140	30	4	6	1
Millet	1/2 cup	207	41	2	6	2
Oats	1/2 cup	150	27	4	5	2.5
Quinoa	1/2 cup	111	20	2.6	4	1.8
Rye Bread	1 slice	83	15	1.5	2.6	1
Sorghum	1/2 cup	316	72	6	10	3.5
Spelt	1/2 cup	127	26	4	6	1
Teff	1/2 cup	255	50	6	9	2
Whole Grain Bagels	1 bagel	245	48	2	8	1
Whole Grain Cereal	1 cup	120	25	5	3	1
Whole Grain Crackers	6 crackers	120	20	3	3	2.5

Whole Grain Crackers	6 crackers	120	20	3	3	2.5
Whole Grain English Muffin	1 muffin	130	27	2	5	1
Whole Grain Muffins	1 muffin	180	30	4	5	2
Whole Grain Pancakes	2 pancakes	200	40	3	6	2
Whole Grain Pita	1 pita	170	35	5	6	1
Whole Grain Tortillas	1 tortilla	80	15	2	3	1
Whole Grain Waffles	2 waffles	210	40	3	5	3

Whole Wheat Bread	1 slice	69	12	1.9	2.7	1
Whole Wheat Pasta	1/2 cup	87	17	2	3.5	0.5
Wild Rice	1/2 cup	83	17	0.7	3	0.3

Fruits and Vegetables

Food Name	Portion Size	Calories (kcal)	Carbohydrates (g)	Fiber (g)	Protein (g)	Fat (g)
Apples	1 medium	95	25	4.4	0.5	0.3
Apricots	1 medium	17	3.9	0.7	0.5	0.1
Avocado	1/2 avocado	161	8.5	6.7	2	15

Bananas	1 mediu m	105	27	3.1	1.3	0.4
Beets	1 cup	59	13	3.8	2.2	0.2
Bell Peppers	1 mediu m	24	5.5	2	0.9	0.2
Berries (mixed)	1 cup	84	21	8	1.5	0.5
Blueberrie s	1 cup	84	21	3.6	1.1	0.5
Broccoli	1 cup	55	11	5.1	4.3	0.6
Brussels Sprouts	1 cup	38	8	3.3	3	0.3
Cantaloup e	1 cup	54	13.7	1.3	1.3	0.3
Carrots	1 mediu m	25	6	2.3	0.6	0.1
Cauliflow er	1 cup	25	5	2	2	0.1

Cucumbers	1 medium	45	11	1.5	2	0.3
Eggplant	1 cup	20	5	3	0.8	0.2
Grapes	1 cup	104	27.3	1.4	0.6	0.2
Kale	1 cup	33	6	1.3	2.9	0.5
Mango	1 cup	99	25	3	1.4	0.6
Oranges	1 medium	62	15	3.1	1.2	0.2
Papaya	1 cup	55	14	2.5	0.5	0.2
Pears	1 medium	102	27	5.5	0.6	0.2
Pineapple	1 cup	82	21.6	2.3	0.9	0.2
Raspberries	1 cup	64	14.7	8	1.5	0.8
Spinach	1 cup	7	1.1	0.7	0.9	0.1
Strawberries	1 cup	49	11.7	3	1	0.4

Sweet Potatoes	1 mediu m	103	24		3.8	2.1	0.2
Tomatoes	1 mediu m	22	5.1		1.5	1.1	0.2
Watermel on	1 cup	46	11.5		0.6	0.9	0.2
Zucchini	1 cup	20	4		1	1.2	0.3

Lean Proteins

Food Name	Porti on Size	Calor ies (kcal)	Prote in (g)	F at (g)	Satura ted Fat (g)	Cholest erol (mg)	Sodi um (mg)
Bison	3 oz	152	25	6. 3	2.6	82	61
Bison Burgers	1 patty	152	26	5. 3	2.2	84	62
Chicke n Breast	3 oz	142	26	3. 1	0.9	82	74

Chicken Sausage	1 link	137	15	7	1.9	57	536
Cottage Cheese	1/2 cup	92	13	2.3	1.4	9	459
Crab	3 oz	84	16	1.1	0.2	45	911
Edamame	1/2 cup	120	11	5	0.7	0	8
Eggs	1 large	72	6	4.8	1.6	186	71
Fish (Cod)	3 oz	89	20	0.7	0.2	42	63
Greek Yogurt	1 cup	133	23	0.4	0.3	10	81
Greek Yogurt (Low-fat)	1 cup	154	23	3.8	2.4	13	99
Halibut	3 oz	119	23	2.3	0.4	39	54

Lean Beef (Top Round)	3 oz	153	26	5.7	2.3	75	46
Lean Pork Chops	3 oz	122	22	3.1	1.1	64	55
Lentils	1/2 cup	115	9	0.4	0.1	0	2
Mussels	3 oz	146	18	3.3	0.5	48	335
Pork Tenderloin	3 oz	122	22	3.1	1.1	64	55
Quorn	1/2 cup	90	10	1	0	0	0
Salmon	3 oz	177	24	8	1.3	55	47
Scallops	3 oz	94	20	0.6	0.1	34	358
Seitan	1/2 cup	160	28	2	0	0	0

Shrimp	3 oz	84	18	0.9	0.1	179	131
Skinless Chicken Thighs	3 oz	166	20	9.3	2.6	88	64
Skinless Turkey Bacon	2 slices	70	10	3	0.9	25	352
Tempeh	1/2 cup	160	16	9	1.5	0	15
Tofu	1/2 cup	94	10	5	0.7	0	8
Trout	3 oz	109	19	3.6	0.8	55	41
Turkey Bacon	2 slices	60	4	4.5	1.3	23	376
Turkey Breast	3 oz	135	29	1.5	0.4	74	53

| Veniso n | 3 oz | 134 | 26 | 2. 4 | 1 | | 74 | 69 |

Dairy and Alternatives

Food Name	Po rti on Siz e	Cal orie s (kc al)	Pr ote in (g)	F a t (g)	Satu rate d Fat (g)	Chol ester ol (mg)	Carb ohyd rates (g)	Cal ciu m (m g)
Almond Milk (Unsweete ned)	1 cup	30	1	2 . 5	0.2	0	1	516
Cashew Milk (Unsweete ned)	1 cup	25	0.5	2	0.3	0	1	25
Cheese (Cheddar)	1 oz	113	7	9	5.6	29	0.4	204
Cheese (Cottage, Low-fat)	1/2 cup	81	14	1	0.5	6	3	69

Cheese (Feta)	1 oz	75	4	6	4	25	1	140
Cheese (Low-fat Mozzarella)	1 oz	72	7	4.5	2.8	18	1	207
Cheese (Mozzarella)	1 oz	72	7	4.5	2.8	18	1	207
Cheese (Parmesan)	1 oz	110	10	7	4.5	20	1	331
Cheese (Provolone)	1 oz	98	7	7.7	4.8	19	0.6	213
Cheese (Ricotta, Part-skim)	1/4 cup	100	8	6	4	23	3	337
Cheese (Swiss)	1 oz	106	7	8.5	5.3	26	1.5	224
Coconut Milk	1 cup	50	0	5	4.6	0	1	481

(Unsweete ned)								
Cottage Cheese (Low-fat)	1/2 cup	81	14	1	0.5	6	3	69
Flax Milk (Unsweete ned)	1 cup	25	0	2.5	0.5	0	1	300
Hazelnut Milk (Unsweete ned)	1 cup	110	2	10	0.9	0	2	516
Hemp Milk (Unsweete ned)	1 cup	70	3	5	0.5	0	1	460
Macadamia Milk (Unsweete ned)	1 cup	50	1	5	0.5	0	1	300
Milk (Skim)	1 cup	83	8	0.2	0.1	5	12	299

Oat Milk (Unsweetened)	1 cup	120	3	5	0.5	0	16	350
Rice Milk (Unsweetened)	1 cup	120	1	2	0.4	0	23	283
Soy Milk (Unsweetened)	1 cup	80	7	4	0.5	0	4	300
Yogurt (Flavored, Low-fat)	1 cup	245	12	2.6	1.7	15	45	345
Yogurt (Greek, Flavored, Low-fat)	1 cup	235	15	4	2.5	18	35	275
Yogurt (Greek, Plain, Low-fat)	1 cup	130	23	0	0	10	9	415
Yogurt (Greek,	1 cup	130	23	0	0	10	9	415

Plain, Non-fat)								
Yogurt (Regular, Flavored, Low-fat)	1 cup	245	11	2.6	1.7	15	45	345
Yogurt (Regular, Flavored, Non-fat)	1 cup	225	11	1.9	1.2	8	45	271
Yogurt (Regular, Non-fat)	1 cup	154	13	0.4	0.2	5	17	488
Yogurt (Regular, Plain, Low-fat)	1 cup	154	13	4.1	2.6	12	17	448
Yogurt (Regular, Plain, Non-fat)	1 cup	154	13	0.4	0.2	5	17	488

Fats and Oils

Food Name	Portion Size	Calories (kcal)	Total Fat (g)	Saturated Fat (g)	Monounsaturated Fat (g)	Polyunsaturated Fat (g)	Omega-3 Fatty Acids (g)	Omega-6 Fatty Acids (g)
Almond Butter	2 tbsp	196	18.2	1.4	8.8	6.9	0.1	6.9
Almonds	1 oz	164	14.2	1.1	9.1	3.4	0.1	3.4
Avocado	1/2 avocado	161	15	2.1	9.8	1.9	0.1	2.1
Avocado Oil	1 tbsp	124	14	1.6	9.9	1.8	0.1	1.8
Brazil Nuts	1 oz	186	18.8	4.3	7.1	5.8	0.1	5.8

Butter	1 tbsp	102	11.5	7.3	3.3	0.4	0	0.4
Canola Oil	1 tbsp	124	14	1	7.1	4.6	0.6	3.4
Cashews	1 oz	157	12.4	2.2	6.7	2.2	0.1	2.2
Chia Seeds	1 oz	138	9	1	0.7	6.7	4.9	1.6
Coconut Butter	1 tbsp	105	11.8	10.9	0.5	0.1	0	0.1
Coconut Oil	1 tbsp	121	13.5	11.2	0.8	0.2	0	0.2
Flaxseed Oil	1 tbsp	120	13.6	1.3	1	9.1	7.3	1.8
Flaxseeds	1 tbsp	37	3	0.3	0.5	2.1	1.6	0.4

Ghee	1 tbsp	112	12.7	7.9	3.7	0.5	0	0.5
Hazel nuts	1 oz	176	17	1.3	13.4	2.2	0.1	2.2
Hemp Seeds	1 oz	161	13.8	1.4	1.1	10.7	0.6	10.1
Lard	1 tbsp	115	12.8	5	5.7	1.4	0.1	1.4
Macadamia Nuts	1 oz	204	21.5	3.4	16.5	0.4	0.1	0.4
Olive Oil	1 tbsp	119	13.5	1.9	9.9	1.4	0.1	1.4
Olive Oil (Extra a	1 tbsp	119	13.5	1.9	9.9	1.4	0.1	1.4

Virgin)								
Peanut Butter	2 tbsp	191	16	3.3	6.6	4.5	0.1	4.5
Pecans	1 oz	196	20.4	1.8	11.6	6.1	0.3	5.8
Pine Nuts	1 oz	191	19	1.4	10.7	5.3	0.1	5.3
Pistachios	1 oz	156	12.9	1.6	6.6	3.9	0.1	3.9
Pumpkin Seeds	1 oz	151	13.1	2.3	4.1	5.9	0.1	5.9
Sesame Oil	1 tbsp	120	13.6	1.9	5.4	5.7	0.1	5.7
Sesame Seeds	1 oz	160	14	2.1	6.5	4.7	0.1	4.7

Sunflower Seeds	1 oz	164	14.2	1.5	3.3	8.9	0.1	8.9
Walnuts	1 oz	183	18.3	1.7	2.5	13.4	2.6	10.7

Herbs, Spices, and Seasonings

Food Name	Portion Size	Calories (kcal)	Total Fat (g)	Sodium (mg)	Carbohydrates (g)	Fiber (g)	Protein (g)
Allspice	1 tsp	6	0	0	1.6	0.9	0.1
Basil	1 tbsp	1	0	0	0.1	0.1	0.1
Bay Leaf	1 leaf	2	0	1	0.4	0.2	0.1
Black Pepper	1 tsp	3	0	0	0.8	0.4	0.1
Caraway Seeds	1 tsp	6	0.3	0	1.1	0.6	0.2
Cardamom	1 tsp	6	0.2	0	1.4	0.6	0.1

Cayenne Pepper	1 tsp	6	0.3	1	1.2	0.6	0.3
Chili Powder	1 tsp	8	0.4	1	1.3	0.8	0.4
Cilantro	1 tbsp	0	0	1	0.1	0	0.1
Cinnamon	1 tsp	6	0	0	2.1	1.3	0.1
Coriander	1 tbsp	5	0	1	1.1	0.6	0.3
Cumin	1 tsp	8	0.5	10	0.7	0.2	0.4
Curry Leaves	1 leaf	1	0	0	0.1	0.1	0.1
Curry Powder	1 tsp	8	0.3	3	1.5	1	0.3
Dill	1 tbsp	2	0	2	0.3	0.2	0.1
Garlic Powder	1 tsp	9	0	1	2.2	0.2	0.5
Ginger	1 tsp	2	0	0	0.5	0.1	0

Mustard Powder	1 tsp	6	0.3	0	0.7	0.5	0.3
Nutmeg	1 tsp	12	0.8	0	0.9	0.6	0.1
Oregano	1 tbsp	3	0	1	0.6	0.4	0.2
Paprika	1 tsp	6	0.3	1	1.4	0.7	0.3
Parsley	1 tbsp	1	0	1	0.1	0.1	0.1
Rosemary	1 tbsp	2	0	1	0.3	0.2	0.1
Saffron	1 tsp	2	0	0	0.5	0.1	0
Sage	1 tbsp	6	0	1	1.4	0.8	0.3
Tarragon	1 tbsp	3	0	1	0.6	0.3	0.2
Thyme	1 tbsp	3	0	1	0.6	0.4	0.2
Turmeric	1 tsp	8	0.2	1	1.4	0.2	0.3
Vanilla Extract	1 tsp	12	0	0	0.5	0	0

CHAPTER FIVE
WEEKLY MEAL PLANNING GUIDE

Building Balanced Meals

Building balanced meals is essential for seniors to maintain good health and well-being. As we age, our nutritional needs may change, requiring us to pay closer attention to the composition of our meals to ensure we're getting the necessary nutrients while avoiding excesses that can lead to health issues. A balanced meal typically includes a combination of macronutrients (carbohydrates, proteins, and fats) along with essential vitamins, minerals, and fiber. Let's delve into some key components of building balanced meals for seniors.

1. Macronutrients:

a. Carbohydrates: Carbohydrates are the body's primary source of energy, especially for seniors who may need a steady supply of energy throughout the day. Opt for complex carbohydrates such as whole grains, fruits, and vegetables, which provide sustained energy and are rich in fiber, aiding in digestion and promoting gut health.

b. Proteins: Proteins are crucial for maintaining muscle mass, bone health, and overall strength, which is particularly important for seniors to support mobility and prevent muscle loss. Include lean sources of protein such as poultry, fish, legumes, tofu, and low-fat dairy products in your meals.

c. Fats: Healthy fats play a vital role in nutrient absorption, brain function, and hormone production. Seniors should focus on incorporating sources of unsaturated fats such as olive oil, avocados, nuts, and seeds into their diet while limiting saturated and trans fats found in fried foods and processed snacks.

2. Micronutrients:

a. Vitamins and Minerals: Seniors may have increased nutrient requirements for certain vitamins and minerals, such as vitamin D, calcium, vitamin B12, and potassium. Include a variety of colorful fruits and vegetables in your meals to ensure you're getting a wide range of vitamins and minerals essential for overall health and immune function.

b. Fiber: Adequate fiber intake is crucial for seniors to support digestive health, prevent constipation, and lower the risk of chronic diseases such as heart disease and diabetes. Whole grains, fruits, vegetables, legumes, and nuts are excellent sources of dietary fiber that should be included in balanced meals.

3. Hydration:

Proper hydration is often overlooked but is essential for seniors to maintain optimal health. Dehydration can lead to various health issues, including urinary tract infections, kidney stones, and cognitive impairment. Encourage seniors to drink plenty of water throughout the day and include hydrating foods such as soups, fruits, and vegetables in their meals.

Portion Control Tips for Seniors

Portion control is essential for seniors to maintain a healthy weight, manage blood sugar levels, and prevent overeating, which can strain the digestive system and lead to discomfort. As we age, our metabolism tends to slow down, making portion control even more critical. Here are some practical tips for seniors to practice portion control effectively:

1. Use Smaller Plates and Bowls:

Using smaller plates and bowls can trick the mind into thinking you're eating more than you are, helping to reduce portion sizes without feeling deprived. Opt for salad plates or smaller bowls for meals to avoid overeating.

2. Mindful Eating:

Practice mindful eating by paying attention to hunger and fullness cues, eating slowly, and savoring each bite. Avoid distractions such as watching TV or using electronic devices while eating, as this can lead to mindless overeating.

3. Measure Portions:

Use measuring cups, spoons, or a food scale to portion out foods, especially when cooking at home. This can help you become more aware of appropriate serving sizes and prevent excessive calorie intake.

4. Fill Half Your Plate with Vegetables:

Vegetables are low in calories but high in nutrients and fiber, making them an excellent choice for filling up without consuming excess calories. Aim to fill half your plate with non-starchy vegetables such as leafy greens, broccoli, peppers, and carrots.

5. Be Mindful of Liquid Calories:

Be mindful of liquid calories from beverages such as soda, fruit juice, and alcohol, as these can contribute to excess calorie intake without providing much satiety. Opt for water, herbal tea, or sparkling water with a splash of lemon or lime instead.

6. Practice Portion Distortion:

Seniors should also be aware of portion distortion when dining out or eating pre-packaged meals, as servings tend to be larger than necessary. Consider splitting meals with a dining companion, ordering appetizers or half-portions, or saving half of the meal for later.

7. Listen to Your Body:

Finally, listen to your body's hunger and fullness cues and stop eating when you feel satisfied, even if there is food left on your plate. Avoid the urge to clean your plate out of habit, as this can lead to overeating.

BREAKFAST RECIPES

Veggie Omelette

Ingredients:

- 1 teaspoon olive oil

- 2 large eggs, lightly beaten

- 1/4 cup diced bell peppers

- 1/4 cup diced onions

- 1/4 cup diced tomatoes

- Salt and pepper to taste

- 1 tablespoon chopped fresh parsley (optional)

Prep Time: 10 mins

Cooking Time: 10 mins

Total Time: 20 mins

Servings: 1

Nutrition Facts (per serving):

- Calories: 210

- Fat: 14g

- Saturated fat: 3.5g

- Cholesterol: 370mg

- Sodium: 270mg

- Carbohydrate: 7g

- Protein: 14g

- Fiber: 2g

Instructions:

1. Heat olive oil in a non-stick skillet over medium heat.

2. Add diced bell peppers, onions, and tomatoes to the skillet. Sauté until vegetables are tender, about 5 minutes.

3. Pour beaten eggs over the vegetables in the skillet. Season with salt and pepper.

4. Cook until the eggs are set, about 3-4 minutes.

5. Carefully fold the omelet in half using a spatula.

6. Transfer the omelet to a plate, garnish with chopped parsley if desired, and serve hot.

Berry Yogurt Parfait

Ingredients:

- 1/2 cup plain Greek yogurt

- 1/4 cup granola

- 1/2 cup mixed berries (such as strawberries, blueberries, raspberries)

- 1 tablespoon honey or maple syrup (optional)

Prep Time: 5 mins

Total Time: 5 mins

Servings: 1

Nutrition Facts (per serving):

- Calories: 250

- Fat: 5g

- Saturated fat: 0.5g

- Cholesterol: 10mg

- Sodium: 60mg

- Carbohydrate: 40g

- Protein: 15g

- Fiber: 6g

Instructions:

1. In a serving glass or bowl, layer Greek yogurt, granola, and mixed berries.

2. Drizzle honey or maple syrup over the top if desired.

3. Serve immediately as a nutritious and refreshing breakfast option.

Whole Grain Pancakes

Ingredients:

- 1 cup whole wheat flour

- 1 tablespoon baking powder

- 1 tablespoon honey or maple syrup

- 1 egg

- 1 cup almond milk (or any milk of choice)

- 1 teaspoon vanilla extract

- Cooking spray or oil for greasing the skillet

Prep Time: 10 mins

Cooking Time: 10 mins

Total Time: 20 mins

Servings: 2 (2-3 pancakes per serving)

Nutrition Facts (per serving):

- Calories: 220

- Fat: 4g

- Saturated fat: 0.5g

- Cholesterol: 55mg

- Sodium: 560mg

- Carbohydrate: 40g

- Protein: 8g

- Fiber: 6g

Instructions:

1. In a mixing bowl, whisk together whole wheat flour and baking powder.

2. In a separate bowl, beat the egg and mix in honey or maple syrup, almond milk, and vanilla extract.

3. Pour the wet ingredients into the dry ingredients and stir until just combined. Do not overmix; a few lumps are okay.

4. Heat a non-stick skillet or griddle over medium heat and lightly grease with cooking spray or oil.

5. Pour about 1/4 cup of batter onto the skillet for each pancake.

6. Cook until bubbles form on the surface of the pancake, then flip and cook until golden brown on both sides.

7. Serve warm with your favorite toppings such as fresh fruit, Greek yogurt, or a drizzle of honey.

Avocado Toast with Poached Egg

Ingredients:

- 1 slice whole grain bread, toasted

- 1/2 ripe avocado

- 1 egg

- Salt and pepper to taste

- Red pepper flakes (optional)

- Chopped fresh herbs (such as cilantro or parsley) for garnish

Prep Time: 5 mins

Cooking Time: 5 mins

Total Time: 10 mins

Servings: 1

Nutrition Facts (per serving):

- Calories: 280

- Fat: 18g

- Saturated fat: 3g

- Cholesterol: 185mg

- Sodium: 240mg

- Carbohydrate: 22g

- Protein: 11g

- Fiber: 8g

Instructions:

1. Mash the ripe avocado with a fork and spread it evenly on the toasted whole-grain bread.

2. Fill a small saucepan with water and bring it to a gentle simmer over medium heat.

3. Crack the egg into a small bowl or ramekin.

4. Carefully slide the egg into the simmering water and poach for about 3-4 minutes, or until the white is set but the yolk is still runny.

5. Remove the poached egg with a slotted spoon and place it on top of the avocado toast.

6. Season with salt, pepper, and red pepper flakes if desired.

7. Garnish with chopped fresh herbs and serve immediately.

Greek Yogurt Smoothie Bowl

Ingredients:

- 1/2 cup plain Greek yogurt

- 1/2 cup mixed berries (such as strawberries, blueberries, raspberries)

- 1/2 ripe banana, sliced

- 1 tablespoon honey or maple syrup

- 1 tablespoon almond butter (or peanut butter)

- 1/4 cup granola

- Chia seeds or flaxseeds for topping (optional)

Prep Time: 5 mins

Total Time: 5 mins

Servings: 1

Nutrition Facts (per serving):

- Calories: 350

- Fat: 10g

- Saturated fat: 1g

- Cholesterol: 10mg

- Sodium: 110mg

- Carbohydrate: 55g

- Protein: 15g

- Fiber: 8g

Instructions:

1. In a blender, combine Greek yogurt, mixed berries, sliced banana, honey or maple syrup, and almond butter.

2. Blend until smooth and creamy, adding a splash of almond milk if needed to reach your desired consistency.

3. Pour the smoothie into a bowl and top with granola and chia seeds or flaxseeds if desired.

4. Serve immediately and enjoy this nutritious and satisfying breakfast option.

Spinach and Feta Egg Muffins

Ingredients:

- 6 large eggs

- 1/4 cup diced bell peppers

- 1/4 cup diced onions

- 1 cup chopped fresh spinach

- 1/4 cup crumbled feta cheese

- Salt and pepper to taste

- Cooking spray or oil for greasing muffin tin

Prep Time: 10 mins

Cooking Time: 20 mins

Total Time: 30 mins

Servings: 6 muffins

Nutrition Facts (per serving - 1 muffin):

- Calories: 90

- Fat: 6g

- Saturated fat: 2g

- Cholesterol: 185mg

- Sodium: 160mg

- Carbohydrate: 2g

- Protein: 7g

- Fiber: 1g

Instructions:

1. Preheat the oven to 350°F (175°C) and grease a muffin tin with cooking spray or oil.

2. In a mixing bowl, beat the eggs and season with salt and pepper.

3. Stir in diced bell peppers, onions, chopped spinach, and crumbled feta cheese until well combined.

4. Pour the egg mixture into the prepared muffin tin, filling each cup about 3/4 full.

5. Bake in the preheated oven for 18-20 minutes, or until the egg muffins are set and slightly golden on top.

6. Allow the egg muffins to cool slightly before removing them from the muffin tin.

7. Serve warm or at room temperature as a convenient and protein-packed breakfast option.

Quinoa Breakfast Bowl

Ingredients:

- 1/2 cup cooked quinoa

- 1/4 cup plain Greek yogurt

- 1/4 cup mixed berries (such as strawberries, blueberries, raspberries)

- 1 tablespoon honey or maple syrup

- 1 tablespoon almond slices or chopped nuts

- 1 teaspoon chia seeds or ground flaxseeds

- Dash of cinnamon (optional)

Prep Time: 5 mins

Total Time: 5 mins

Servings: 1

Nutrition Facts (per serving):

- Calories: 280

- Fat: 8g

- Saturated fat: 1g

- Cholesterol: 5mg

- Sodium: 25mg

- Carbohydrate: 45g

- Protein: 10g

- Fiber: 6g

Instructions:

1. In a serving bowl, layer cooked quinoa, plain Greek yogurt, and mixed berries.

2. Drizzle honey or maple syrup over the top.

3. Sprinkle almond slices or chopped nuts and chia seeds or ground flaxseeds on top.

4. Add a dash of cinnamon if desired for extra flavor.

5. Serve immediately as a wholesome and satisfying breakfast option.

Sweet Potato Hash with Turkey Sausage

Ingredients:

- 1 medium sweet potato, peeled and diced

- 2 turkey sausage links, sliced

- 1/4 cup diced bell peppers

- 1/4 cup diced onions

- 1 tablespoon olive oil

- Salt and pepper to taste

- Chopped fresh parsley for garnish (optional)

Prep Time: 10 mins

Cooking Time: 20 mins

Total Time: 30 mins

Servings: 2

Nutrition Facts (per serving):

- Calories: 280

- Fat: 12g

- Saturated fat: 2.5g

- Cholesterol: 50mg

- Sodium: 420mg

- Carbohydrate: 28g

- Protein: 15g

- Fiber: 4g

Instructions:

1. Heat olive oil in a skillet over medium heat.

2. Add diced sweet potatoes to the skillet and cook until tender, about 8-10 minutes.

3. Add sliced turkey sausage, diced bell peppers, and diced onions to the skillet. Cook until sausage is browned and vegetables are tender about 6-8 minutes.

4. Season with salt and pepper to taste.

5. Garnish with chopped fresh parsley if desired before serving.

6. Serve hot as a flavourful and nutritious breakfast option.

Cottage Cheese and Fruit Bowl

Ingredients:

- 1/2 cup low-fat cottage cheese

- 1/2 cup mixed fruit (such as diced apples, sliced bananas, berries)

- 1 tablespoon chopped nuts (such as almonds, walnuts, or pecans)

- 1 tablespoon honey or maple syrup

- Dash of cinnamon (optional)

Prep Time: 5 mins

Total Time: 5 mins

Servings: 1

Nutrition Facts (per serving):

- Calories: 250

- Fat: 8g

- Saturated fat: 1.5g

- Cholesterol: 10mg

- Sodium: 400mg

- Carbohydrate: 30g

- Protein: 15g

- Fiber: 4g

Instructions:

1. In a serving bowl, layer low-fat cottage cheese and mixed fruit.

2. Drizzle honey or maple syrup over the top.

3. Sprinkle chopped nuts on top for added crunch and protein.

4. Add a dash of cinnamon if desired for extra flavor.

5. Serve immediately as a delicious and protein-rich breakfast option.

Breakfast Burrito

Ingredients:

- 2 large eggs, lightly beaten

- 2 whole grain tortillas

- 1/4 cup diced bell peppers

- 1/4 cup diced onions

- 1/4 cup black beans, drained and rinsed

- 1/4 cup shredded cheddar cheese

- Salsa and sliced avocado for serving (optional)

Prep Time: 10 mins

Cooking Time: 10 mins

Total Time: 20 mins

Servings: 2

Nutrition Facts (per serving):

- Calories: 320

- Fat: 15g

- Saturated fat: 5g

- Cholesterol: 215mg

- Sodium: 530mg

- Carbohydrate: 28g

- Protein: 18g

- Fiber: 6g

Instructions:

1. Heat a non-stick skillet over medium heat.

2. Add diced bell peppers and onions to the skillet and cook until softened about 3-4 minutes.

3. Add beaten eggs to the skillet and scramble until cooked through about 2-3 minutes.

4. Warm whole grain tortillas in the microwave or on a skillet for a few seconds.

5. Divide scrambled eggs, black beans, and shredded cheddar cheese between the tortillas.

6. Roll up the tortillas into burritos, folding in the sides to enclose the filling.

7. Serve with salsa and sliced avocado on the side if desired.

8. Enjoy this satisfying and protein-packed breakfast on the
    go.

LUNCH RECIPES

Quinoa Salad with Grilled Chicken

Ingredients:

- 1 cup quinoa, rinsed

- 2 cups water or low-sodium chicken broth

- 2 boneless, skinless chicken breasts

- 1 tablespoon olive oil

- Salt and pepper to taste

- 1/2 cup diced cucumber

- 1/2 cup diced tomatoes

- 1/4 cup diced red onion

- 1/4 cup chopped fresh parsley

- 2 tablespoons lemon juice

- 1 tablespoon balsamic vinegar

Prep Time: 10 mins

Cooking Time: 20 mins

Total Time: 30 mins

Servings: 2

Nutrition Facts (per serving):

- Calories: 420

- Fat: 12g

- Saturated fat: 2g

- Cholesterol: 80mg

- Sodium: 150mg

- Carbohydrate: 45g

- Protein: 35g

- Fiber: 6g

Instructions:

1. In a medium saucepan, combine quinoa and water or chicken broth. Bring to a boil, then reduce heat to low, cover, and simmer for 15-20 minutes, or until quinoa is tender and liquid is absorbed. Remove from heat and let it cool.

2. Meanwhile, preheat the grill or grill pan over medium-high heat. Brush chicken breasts with olive oil and season with salt and pepper. Grill for 6-8 minutes per side, or until cooked through. Let chicken rest for a few minutes, then slice into strips.

3. In a large bowl, combine cooked quinoa, diced cucumber, tomatoes, red onion, and chopped parsley.

4. In a small bowl, whisk together lemon juice and balsamic vinegar to make the dressing.

5. Add grilled chicken strips to the quinoa salad, then drizzle with the dressing and toss to coat.

6. Divide the salad between plates and serve immediately as a nutritious and satisfying lunch option.

Turkey and Avocado Wrap

Ingredients:

- 2 whole grain tortillas

- 4 slices deli turkey breast

- 1/2 avocado, sliced

- 1/4 cup shredded lettuce

- 1/4 cup diced tomatoes

- 2 tablespoons hummus

- Salt and pepper to taste

Prep Time: 10 mins

Total Time: 10 mins

Servings: 2

Nutrition Facts (per serving):

- Calories: 300

- Fat: 12g

- Saturated fat: 2g

- Cholesterol: 25mg

- Sodium: 600mg

- Carbohydrate: 35g

- Protein: 15g

- Fiber: 8g

Instructions:

1. Lay out the whole-grain tortillas on a flat surface.

2. Spread hummus evenly over each tortilla.

3. Arrange turkey breast slices, avocado slices, shredded lettuce, and diced tomatoes on top of the hummus.

4. Season with salt and pepper to taste.

5. Roll up the tortillas tightly into wraps, folding in the sides to enclose the filling.

6. Slice the wraps in half diagonally and serve immediately, or wrap in foil for a convenient on-the-go lunch option.

Salmon and Quinoa Bowl

Ingredients:

- 2 salmon fillets

- 1 tablespoon olive oil

- Salt and pepper to taste

- 1 cup cooked quinoa

- 1 cup steamed broccoli florets

- 1/2 cup shredded carrots

- 1/4 cup sliced almonds

- Lemon wedges for serving

Prep Time: 10 mins

Cooking Time: 15 mins

Total Time: 25 mins

Servings: 2

Nutrition Facts (per serving):

- Calories: 400

- Fat: 20g

- Saturated fat: 3g

- Cholesterol: 50mg

- Sodium: 300mg

- Carbohydrate: 30g

- Protein: 30g

- Fiber: 8g

Instructions:

1. Preheat oven to 400°F (200°C). Line a baking sheet with parchment paper.

2. Place salmon fillets on the prepared baking sheet. Drizzle with olive oil and season with salt and pepper.

3. Bake salmon in the preheated oven for 12-15 minutes, or until cooked through and flaky.

4. Meanwhile, divide cooked quinoa, steamed broccoli florets, and shredded carrots between serving bowls.

5. Top each bowl with a baked salmon fillet.

6. Sprinkle sliced almonds over the bowls and serve with lemon wedges on the side.

7. Enjoy this nutritious and flavourful salmon and quinoa bowl for a satisfying lunch.

Chickpea and Spinach Salad

Ingredients:

- 1 can (15 oz) chickpeas, drained and rinsed

- 2 cups fresh baby spinach leaves

- 1/4 cup sliced red onion

- 1/4 cup diced cucumber

- 1/4 cup diced tomatoes

- 2 tablespoons crumbled feta cheese

- 2 tablespoons lemon juice

- 1 tablespoon extra-virgin olive oil

- 1 teaspoon dried oregano

- Salt and pepper to taste

Prep Time: 10 mins

Total Time: 10 mins

Servings: 2

Nutrition Facts (per serving):

- Calories: 250

- Fat: 10g

- Saturated fat: 2g

- Cholesterol: 5mg

- Sodium: 300mg

- Carbohydrate: 30g

- Protein: 10g

- Fiber: 8g

Instructions:

1. In a large bowl, combine chickpeas, baby spinach leaves, sliced red onion, diced cucumber, diced tomatoes, and crumbled feta cheese.

2. In a small bowl, whisk together lemon juice, olive oil, dried oregano, salt, and pepper to make the dressing.

3. Drizzle the dressing over the salad and toss to coat evenly.

4. Divide the salad between plates and serve immediately as a light and refreshing lunch option.

Vegetable Stir-Fry with Tofu

Ingredients:

- 1 block (14 oz) firm tofu, pressed and cubed

- 2 tablespoons soy sauce

- 1 tablespoon sesame oil

- 1 tablespoon cornstarch

- 1 tablespoon vegetable oil

- 2 cups mixed vegetables (such as bell peppers, broccoli, carrots, snap peas)

- 2 cloves garlic, minced

- 1 teaspoon grated fresh ginger

- Cooked brown rice for serving

Prep Time: 15 mins

Cooking Time: 15 mins

Total Time: 30 mins

Servings: 2

Nutrition Facts (per serving):

- Calories: 350

- Fat: 18g

- Saturated fat: 3g

- Cholesterol: 0mg

- Sodium: 600mg

- Carbohydrate: 25g

- Protein: 20g

- Fiber: 6g

Instructions:

1. In a shallow dish, whisk together soy sauce, sesame oil, and cornstarch. Add cubed tofu and toss to coat. Let marinate for 10 minutes.

2. Heat vegetable oil in a large skillet or wok over medium-high heat. Add marinated tofu cubes and cook until golden brown on all sides, about 5-7 minutes. Remove tofu from the skillet and set aside.

3. In the same skillet, add mixed vegetables, minced garlic, and grated ginger. Stir-fry for 5-7 minutes, or until vegetables are tender-crisp.

4. Return cooked tofu to the skillet and toss with the vegetables.

5. Serve vegetable stir-fry with tofu over cooked brown rice and enjoy a flavourful and nutritious lunch.

Turkey and Vegetable Stir-Fry

Ingredients:

- 2 turkey cutlets, thinly sliced
- 2 tablespoons soy sauce
- 1 tablespoon sesame oil
- 1 tablespoon cornstarch
- 1 tablespoon vegetable oil
- 2 cups mixed vegetables (such as bell peppers, broccoli, carrots, snow peas)
- 2 cloves garlic, minced
- 1 teaspoon grated fresh ginger
- Cooked brown rice for serving

Prep Time: 15 mins

Cooking Time: 15 mins

Total Time: 30 mins

Servings: 2

Nutrition Facts (per serving):

- Calories: 320
- Fat: 12g

- Saturated fat: 2g

- Cholesterol: 70mg

- Sodium: 700mg

- Carbohydrate: 25g

- Protein: 25g

- Fiber: 6g

Instructions:

1. In a shallow dish, whisk together soy sauce, sesame oil, and cornstarch. Add sliced turkey cutlets and toss to coat. Let marinate for 10 minutes.

2. Heat vegetable oil in a large skillet or wok over medium-high heat. Add marinated turkey slices and cook until browned and cooked through about 5-7 minutes. Remove turkey from skillet and set aside.

3. In the same skillet, add mixed vegetables, minced garlic, and grated ginger. Stir-fry for 5-7 minutes, or until vegetables are tender-crisp.

4. Return the cooked turkey to the skillet and toss it with the vegetables.

5. Serve turkey and vegetable stir-fry over cooked brown rice for a delicious and healthy lunch option.

Mediterranean Chickpea Salad

Ingredients:

- 1 can (15 oz) chickpeas, drained and rinsed
- 1 cup diced cucumber
- 1 cup halved cherry tomatoes
- 1/4 cup diced red onion
- 1/4 cup chopped fresh parsley
- 2 tablespoons extra virgin olive oil
- 1 tablespoon lemon juice
- 1 teaspoon dried oregano
- Salt and pepper to taste
- Crumbled feta cheese for garnish (optional)

Prep Time: 10 mins

Total Time: 10 mins

Servings: 2

Nutrition Facts (per serving):

- Calories: 280
- Fat: 14g
- Saturated fat: 2g
- Cholesterol: 0mg

- Sodium: 400mg

- Carbohydrate: 30g

- Protein: 10g

- Fiber: 8g

Instructions:

1. In a large bowl, combine chickpeas, diced cucumber, halved cherry tomatoes, diced red onion, and chopped fresh parsley.

2. In a small bowl, whisk together extra virgin olive oil, lemon juice, dried oregano, salt, and pepper to make the dressing.

3. Drizzle the dressing over the chickpea salad and toss to coat evenly.

4. Garnish with crumbled feta cheese if desired.

5. Serve Mediterranean chickpea salad as a refreshing and nutritious lunch option.

Lentil Soup with Spinach

Ingredients:

- 1 cup dried lentils, rinsed and drained

- 4 cups low-sodium vegetable broth

- 1 tablespoon olive oil

- 1 onion, diced

- 2 carrots, diced

- 2 celery stalks, diced

- 2 cloves garlic, minced

- 1 teaspoon ground cumin

- 1/2 teaspoon smoked paprika

- 1 bay leaf

- 2 cups fresh baby spinach leaves

- Salt and pepper to taste

- Lemon wedges for serving (optional)

Prep Time: 10 mins

Cooking Time: 30 mins

Total Time: 40 mins

Servings: 4

Nutrition Facts (per serving):

- Calories: 250

- Fat: 4g

- Saturated fat: 0.5g

- Cholesterol: 0mg

- Sodium: 500mg

- Carbohydrate: 40g

- Protein: 15g

- Fiber: 15g

Instructions:

1. In a large pot, heat olive oil over medium heat. Add diced onion, carrots, and celery. Cook until vegetables are softened, about 5-7 minutes.

2. Add minced garlic, ground cumin, and smoked paprika to the pot. Cook for another 1-2 minutes, until fragrant.

3. Stir in rinsed lentils, vegetable broth, and bay leaf. Bring to a boil, then reduce heat to low, cover, and simmer for 20-25 minutes, or until lentils are tender.

4. Add fresh baby spinach leaves to the soup and stir until wilted.

5. Season with salt and pepper to taste.

6. Serve lentil soup with spinach hot, with lemon wedges on the side if desired.

Tuna Salad Stuffed Avocado

Ingredients:

- 2 ripe avocados

- 1 can (5 oz) tuna, drained

- 1/4 cup diced red onion

- 1/4 cup diced cucumber

- 1/4 cup diced bell pepper

- 2 tablespoons plain Greek yogurt

- 1 tablespoon lemon juice

- 1 tablespoon chopped fresh parsley

- Salt and pepper to taste

Prep Time: 10 mins

Total Time: 10 mins

Servings: 2

Nutrition Facts (per serving):

- Calories: 320

- Fat: 20g

- Saturated fat: 3g

- Cholesterol: 20mg

- Sodium: 350mg

- Carbohydrate: 20g

- Protein: 20g

- Fiber: 10g

Instructions:

1. Cut avocados in half and remove pits. Scoop out some of the flesh from each half to create a larger cavity for the filling, leaving a border around the edges.

2. In a medium bowl, combine drained tuna, diced red onion, diced cucumber, diced bell pepper, plain Greek yogurt, lemon juice, chopped fresh parsley, salt, and pepper.

3. Spoon the tuna salad mixture into the avocado halves, dividing evenly.

4. Serve tuna salad stuffed avocados immediately as a light and satisfying lunch option.

Vegetable and Bean Burrito Bowl

Ingredients:

- 1 cup cooked brown rice

- 1 can (15 oz) black beans, drained and rinsed

- 1 cup diced bell peppers

- 1 cup diced tomatoes

- 1/2 cup shredded lettuce

- 1/4 cup diced red onion

- 1/4 cup chopped fresh cilantro

- 1 avocado, sliced

- Lime wedges for serving

- Salsa and Greek yogurt for topping (optional)

Prep Time: 10 mins

Total Time: 10 mins

Servings: 2

Nutrition Facts (per serving):

- Calories: 380

- Fat: 12g

- Saturated fat: 2g

- Cholesterol: 0mg

- Sodium: 450mg

- Carbohydrate: 60g

- Protein: 15g

- Fiber: 15g

Instructions:

1. Divide cooked brown rice between serving bowls.

2. Top rice with black beans, diced bell peppers, diced tomatoes, shredded lettuce, diced red onion, and chopped fresh cilantro.

3. Arrange avocado slices on top of the bowl.

4. Serve vegetable and bean burrito bowls with lime wedges on the side.

5. Add salsa and Greek yogurt as desired for extra flavor.

6. Enjoy this nutritious and flavourful burrito bowl for lunch.

DINNER RECIPES

Grilled Salmon with Lemon-Dill Sauce

Ingredients:

- 2 salmon fillets

- 1 tablespoon olive oil

- Salt and pepper to taste

- 1 lemon, thinly sliced

- Fresh dill for garnish

For the Lemon-Dill Sauce:

- 1/4 cup plain Greek yogurt

- 1 tablespoon lemon juice

- 1 tablespoon chopped fresh dill

- 1 teaspoon Dijon mustard

- Salt and pepper to taste

Prep Time: 10 mins

Cooking Time: 10 mins

Total Time: 20 mins

Servings: 2

Nutrition Facts (per serving):

- Calories: 300

- Fat: 15g

- Saturated fat: 2g

- Cholesterol: 80mg

- Sodium: 250mg

- Carbohydrate: 2g

- Protein: 35g

Instructions:

1. Preheat the grill to medium-high heat.

2. Brush salmon fillets with olive oil and season with salt and pepper.

3. Place lemon slices on top of each salmon fillet.

4. Grill salmon for 4-5 minutes per side, or until cooked through and flaky.

5. Meanwhile, prepare the lemon-dill sauce by combining Greek yogurt, lemon juice, chopped fresh dill, Dijon mustard, salt, and pepper in a bowl. Mix well.

6. Serve grilled salmon with lemon-dill sauce drizzled over the top and garnished with fresh dill sprigs.

Vegetable Stir-Fry with Tofu

Ingredients:

- 1 block (14 oz) firm tofu, cubed

- 2 tablespoons soy sauce

- 1 tablespoon sesame oil

- 1 tablespoon cornstarch

- 1 tablespoon vegetable oil

- 2 cups mixed vegetables (such as bell peppers, broccoli, carrots, snap peas)

- 2 cloves garlic, minced

- 1 teaspoon grated fresh ginger

- Cooked brown rice for serving

Prep Time: 15 mins

Cooking Time: 15 mins

Total Time: 30 mins

Servings: 2

Nutrition Facts (per serving):

- Calories: 350

- Fat: 18g

- Saturated fat: 3g

- Cholesterol: 0mg

- Sodium: 600mg

- Carbohydrate: 25g

- Protein: 20g

- Fiber: 6g

Instructions:

1. In a shallow dish, combine cubed tofu, soy sauce, sesame oil, and cornstarch. Toss to coat tofu evenly.

2. Heat vegetable oil in a large skillet or wok over medium-high heat.

3. Add tofu cubes to the skillet and cook until golden brown on all sides, about 5-7 minutes. Remove tofu from the skillet and set aside.

4. In the same skillet, add mixed vegetables, minced garlic, and grated ginger. Stir-fry for 5-7 minutes, or until vegetables are tender-crisp.

5. Return cooked tofu to the skillet and toss with the vegetables until heated through.

6. Serve vegetable stir-fry with tofu over cooked brown rice for a delicious and nutritious dinner.

Mediterranean Stuffed Bell Peppers

Ingredients:

- 2 large bell peppers, halved and seeds removed

- 1 cup cooked quinoa

- 1 can (15 oz) chickpeas, drained and rinsed

- 1/2 cup diced tomatoes

- 1/4 cup chopped kalamata olives

- 1/4 cup crumbled feta cheese

- 1 tablespoon olive oil

- 1 teaspoon dried oregano

- Salt and pepper to taste

- Fresh parsley for garnish

Prep Time: 15 mins

Cooking Time: 30 mins

Total Time: 45 mins

Servings: 2 (4 halves)

Nutrition Facts (per serving):

- Calories: 350

- Fat: 12g

- Saturated fat: 3g

- Cholesterol: 10mg

- Sodium: 400mg

- Carbohydrate: 45g

- Protein: 15g

- Fiber: 10g

Instructions:

1. Preheat oven to 375°F (190°C). Line a baking dish with parchment paper.

2. In a large bowl, combine cooked quinoa, chickpeas, diced tomatoes, chopped kalamata olives, crumbled feta cheese, olive oil, dried oregano, salt, and pepper.

3. Stuff each bell pepper half with the quinoa mixture and place them in the prepared baking dish.

4. Cover the dish with foil and bake in the preheated oven for 25-30 minutes, or until bell peppers are tender.

5. Remove the foil and bake for an additional 5 minutes to brown the tops of the peppers.

6. Garnish stuffed bell peppers with fresh parsley before serving.

Lemon Herb Chicken with Roasted Vegetables

Ingredients:

- 2 boneless, skinless chicken breasts

- 2 tablespoons olive oil

- 2 cloves garlic, minced

- 1 tablespoon chopped fresh rosemary

- 1 tablespoon chopped fresh thyme

- 1 tablespoon lemon zest

- Salt and pepper to taste

- 2 cups mixed vegetables (such as carrots, potatoes, Brussels sprouts)

- Lemon wedges for serving

Prep Time: 15 mins

Cooking Time: 25 mins

Total Time: 40 mins

Servings: 2

Nutrition Facts (per serving):

- Calories: 320

- Fat: 15g

- Saturated fat: 2g

- Cholesterol: 80mg

- Sodium: 300mg

- Carbohydrate: 20g

- Protein: 30g

- Fiber: 6g

Instructions:

1. Preheat oven to 400°F (200°C). Line a baking sheet with parchment paper.

2. In a small bowl, combine olive oil, minced garlic, chopped fresh rosemary, chopped fresh thyme, lemon zest, salt, and pepper to make a marinade.

3. Place chicken breasts in a shallow dish and coat them with the marinade. Let marinate for 10-15 minutes.

4. Meanwhile, prepare mixed vegetables by chopping them into bite-sized pieces.

5. Arrange marinated chicken breasts and mixed vegetables on the prepared baking sheet.

6. Roast in the preheated oven for 20-25 minutes, or until chicken is cooked through and vegetables are tender.

7. Serve lemon herb chicken with roasted vegetables, with lemon wedges on the side.

Lentil and Vegetable Curry

Ingredients:

- 1 cup dried green lentils, rinsed and drained

- 4 cups low-sodium vegetable broth

- 1 tablespoon olive oil

- 1 onion, diced

- 2 carrots, diced

- 2 potatoes, diced

- 2 cups cauliflower florets

- 1 can (14 oz) diced tomatoes

- 1 can (14 oz) coconut milk

- 2 tablespoons curry powder

- Salt and pepper to taste

- Fresh cilantro for garnish

- Cooked brown rice for serving

Prep Time: 15 mins

Cooking Time: 30 mins

Total Time: 45 mins

Servings: 4

Nutrition Facts (per serving):

- Calories: 380

- Fat: 15g

- Saturated fat: 10g

- Cholesterol: 0mg

- Sodium: 500mg

- Carbohydrate: 45g

- Protein: 15g

- Fiber: 12g

Instructions:

1. In a large pot, heat olive oil over medium heat. Add diced onion and cook until softened about 5 minutes.

2. Add diced carrots, diced potatoes, and cauliflower florets to the pot. Cook for another 5 minutes, stirring occasionally.

3. Stir in rinsed lentils, low-sodium vegetable broth, diced tomatoes, coconut milk, and curry powder.

4. Bring the mixture to a boil, then reduce heat to low, cover, and simmer for 20-25 minutes, or until lentils and vegetables are tender.

5. Season with salt and pepper to taste.

6. Serve lentil and vegetable curry over cooked brown rice, garnished with fresh cilantro. Enjoy this hearty and flavourful curry for dinner.

Baked Cod with Herbed Quinoa

Ingredients:

- 2 cod fillets

- 1 tablespoon olive oil

- 1 tablespoon lemon juice

- 1 teaspoon dried thyme

- 1 teaspoon dried parsley

- Salt and pepper to taste

- 1 cup cooked quinoa

- 1 tablespoon chopped fresh parsley

- Lemon wedges for serving

Prep Time: 10 mins

Cooking Time: 20 mins

Total Time: 30 mins

Servings: 2

Nutrition Facts (per serving):

- Calories: 250

- Fat: 8g

- Saturated fat: 1g

- Cholesterol: 50mg

- Sodium: 200mg

- Carbohydrate: 20g

- Protein: 25g

- Fiber: 3g

Instructions:

1. Preheat oven to 400°F (200°C). Line a baking sheet with parchment paper.

2. Place cod fillets on the prepared baking sheet.

3. In a small bowl, whisk together olive oil, lemon juice, dried thyme, dried parsley, salt, and pepper.

4. Brush the herb mixture over the cod fillets.

5. Bake in the preheated oven for 15-20 minutes, or until the cod is opaque and flakes easily with a fork.

6. While the cod is baking, fluff cooked quinoa with a fork and stir in chopped fresh parsley.

7. Serve baked cod with herbed quinoa and lemon wedges on the side.

Turkey and Vegetable Skillet

Ingredients:

- 1 lb ground turkey

- 1 tablespoon olive oil

- 1 onion, diced

- 2 cloves garlic, minced

- 1 bell pepper, diced

- 1 zucchini, diced

- 1 cup cherry tomatoes, halved

- 1 teaspoon Italian seasoning

- Salt and pepper to taste

- Fresh basil for garnish

Prep Time: 10 mins

Cooking Time: 20 mins

Total Time: 30 mins

Servings: 4

Nutrition Facts (per serving):

- Calories: 280

- Fat: 15g

- Saturated fat: 3g

- Cholesterol: 80mg

- Sodium: 300mg

- Carbohydrate: 10g

- Protein: 25g

- Fiber: 3g

Instructions:

1. Heat olive oil in a large skillet over medium heat. Add diced onion and cook until softened about 5 minutes.

2. Add minced garlic and ground turkey to the skillet. Cook until turkey is browned and cooked through, breaking it up with a spoon as it cooks.

3. Stir in diced bell pepper, diced zucchini, halved cherry tomatoes, Italian seasoning, salt, and pepper. Cook for another 5-7 minutes, or until vegetables are tender.

4. Garnish turkey and vegetable skillet with fresh basil leaves before serving.

Quinoa Stuffed Bell Peppers

Ingredients:

- 2 large bell peppers, halved and seeds removed

- 1 cup cooked quinoa

- 1 can (15 oz) black beans, drained and rinsed

- 1 cup corn kernels (fresh or frozen)

- 1/2 cup diced tomatoes

- 1/4 cup diced red onion

- 1/4 cup chopped fresh cilantro

- 1 teaspoon ground cumin

- Salt and pepper to taste

- Shredded cheddar cheese for topping (optional)

Prep Time: 15 mins

Cooking Time: 30 mins

Total Time: 45 mins

Servings: 2 (4 halves)

Nutrition Facts (per serving):

- Calories: 320

- Fat: 5g

- Saturated fat: 1g

- Cholesterol: 0mg

- Sodium: 300mg

- Carbohydrate: 55g

- Protein: 15g

- Fiber: 12g

Instructions:

1. Preheat oven to 375°F (190°C). Line a baking dish with parchment paper.

2. In a large bowl, combine cooked quinoa, black beans, corn kernels, diced tomatoes, diced red onion, chopped fresh cilantro, ground cumin, salt, and pepper.

3. Stuff each bell pepper half with the quinoa mixture and place them in the prepared baking dish.

4. Cover the dish with foil and bake in the preheated oven for 25-30 minutes, or until bell peppers are tender.

5. Remove foil and sprinkle shredded cheddar cheese on top of each stuffed bell pepper, if desired. Bake for an additional 5 minutes, or until cheese is melted and bubbly.

6. Serve quinoa stuffed bell peppers hot as a wholesome and satisfying dinner option.

Chicken and Vegetable Curry

Ingredients:

- 2 boneless, skinless chicken breasts, cubed

- 1 tablespoon olive oil

- 1 onion, diced

- 2 cloves garlic, minced

- 1 bell pepper, diced

- 1 zucchini, diced

- 1 cup diced tomatoes

- 1 can (14 oz) coconut milk

- 2 tablespoons curry powder

- Salt and pepper to taste

- Cooked brown rice for serving

Prep Time: 15 mins

Cooking Time: 25 mins

Total Time: 40 mins

Servings: 2

Nutrition Facts (per serving):

- Calories: 350

- Fat: 15g

- Saturated fat: 10g

- Cholesterol: 70mg

- Sodium: 400mg

- Carbohydrate: 25g

- Protein: 30g

- Fiber: 6g

Instructions:

1. Heat olive oil in a large skillet over medium heat. Add diced onion and cook until softened about 5 minutes.

2. Add minced garlic and cubed chicken breast to the skillet. Cook until chicken is browned on all sides, about 5 minutes.

3. Stir in diced bell pepper, diced zucchini, and diced tomatoes. Cook for another 5 minutes, or until vegetables are tender.

4. Pour in coconut milk and sprinkle curry powder over the mixture. Stir well to combine.

5. Simmer chicken and vegetable curry for 10-15 minutes, or until chicken is cooked through and flavors are well combined.

6. Season with salt and pepper to taste.

7. Serve chicken and vegetable curry over cooked brown rice
   for a delicious and satisfying dinner.

Shrimp and Vegetable Stir-Fry

Ingredients:

- 1 lb shrimp, peeled and deveined

- 2 tablespoons soy sauce

- 1 tablespoon sesame oil

- 1 tablespoon cornstarch

- 1 tablespoon vegetable oil

- 2 cups mixed vegetables (such as broccoli, snap peas,
  carrots)

- 2 cloves garlic, minced

- 1 teaspoon grated fresh ginger

- Cooked brown rice for serving

Prep Time: 15 mins

Cooking Time: 15 mins

Total Time: 30 mins

Servings: 2

Nutrition Facts (per serving):

- Calories: 300

- Fat: 10g

- Saturated fat: 2g

- Cholesterol: 200mg

- Sodium: 700mg

- Carbohydrate: 20g

- Protein: 30g

- Fiber: 4g

Instructions:

1. In a shallow dish, combine peeled and deveined shrimp with soy sauce, sesame oil, and cornstarch. Toss to coat shrimp evenly.

2. Heat vegetable oil in a large skillet or wok over medium-high heat.

3. Add marinated shrimp to the skillet and cook until pink and opaque, about 2-3 minutes per side. Remove shrimp from the skillet and set aside.

4. In the same skillet, add mixed vegetables, minced garlic, and grated ginger. Stir-fry for 5-7 minutes, or until vegetables are tender-crisp.

5. Return cooked shrimp to the skillet and toss with the vegetables until heated through.

6. Serve shrimp and vegetable stir-fry over cooked brown rice for a quick and flavourful dinner option.

SNACKS AND APPETIZER RECIPES

Avocado and White Bean Dip

Ingredients:

- 1 ripe avocado

- 1 can (15 oz) white beans, drained and rinsed

- 1 clove garlic, minced

- 2 tablespoons fresh lemon juice

- 1 tablespoon olive oil

- Salt and pepper to taste

- Pinch of cayenne pepper (optional)

- Fresh cilantro for garnish

- Whole grain crackers or vegetable sticks for serving

Prep Time: 10 mins

Total Time: 10 mins

Servings: 4

Nutrition Facts (per serving):

- Calories: 120

- Fat: 6g

- Saturated fat: 1g

- Cholesterol: 0mg

- Sodium: 200mg

- Carbohydrate: 13g

- Protein: 4g

- Fiber: 5g

Instructions:

1. In a food processor, combine ripe avocado, white beans, minced garlic, fresh lemon juice, olive oil, salt, pepper, and cayenne pepper (if using).

2. Blend until smooth and creamy, scraping down the sides as needed.

3. Transfer the dip to a serving bowl and garnish with fresh cilantro.

4. Serve avocado and white bean dip with whole grain crackers or vegetable sticks for a healthy and satisfying snack.

Greek Yogurt and Berry Parfait

Ingredients:

- 1 cup plain Greek yogurt

- 1/2 cup mixed berries (such as strawberries, blueberries, raspberries)

- 1 tablespoon honey or maple syrup

- 1/4 cup granola

- Fresh mint leaves for garnish (optional)

Prep Time: 5 mins

Total Time: 5 mins

Servings: 1

Nutrition Facts (per serving):

- Calories: 250

- Fat: 5g

- Saturated fat: 0.5g

- Cholesterol: 10mg

- Sodium: 50mg

- Carbohydrate: 35g

- Protein: 18g

- Fiber: 5g

Instructions:

1. In a serving glass or bowl, layer plain Greek yogurt, mixed berries, and honey or maple syrup.

2. Sprinkle granola on top of the yogurt and berry mixture.

3. Garnish with fresh mint leaves if desired.

4. Serve Greek yogurt and berry parfait immediately as a nutritious and refreshing snack option.

Hummus and Veggie Platter

Ingredients:

- 1 cup hummus (store-bought or homemade)
- Assorted fresh vegetables (such as carrots, cucumber, bell peppers, cherry tomatoes)
- Whole grain pita bread or crackers

Prep Time: 10 mins

Total Time: 10 mins

Servings: 4

Nutrition Facts (per serving):

- Calories: 150
- Fat: 7g
- Saturated fat: 1g
- Cholesterol: 0mg
- Sodium: 250mg
- Carbohydrate: 18g
- Protein: 6g
- Fiber: 6g

Instructions:

1. Arrange the hummus in the center of a serving platter or plate.

2. Surround the hummus with assorted fresh vegetables and whole-grain pita bread or crackers.

3. Serve hummus and veggie platter as a nutritious and satisfying appetizer or snack option.

Cucumber and Smoked Salmon Roll-Ups

Ingredients:

- 1 large cucumber

- 4 oz smoked salmon

- 4 oz cream cheese

- Fresh dill for garnish

Prep Time: 10 mins

Total Time: 10 mins

Servings: 4

Nutrition Facts (per serving):

- Calories: 120

- Fat: 8g

- Saturated fat: 4g

- Cholesterol: 25mg

- Sodium: 300mg

- Carbohydrate: 3g

- Protein: 10g

- Fiber: 1g

Instructions:

1. Use a vegetable peeler to slice the cucumber lengthwise into thin strips.

2. Spread a thin layer of cream cheese on each cucumber strip.

3. Place a slice of smoked salmon on top of the cream cheese.

4. Roll up the cucumber strip with the smoked salmon inside.

5. Secure each roll-up with a toothpick if necessary.

6. Garnish cucumber and smoked salmon roll-ups with fresh dill before serving.

Stuffed Mini Bell Peppers

Ingredients:

- 12 mini bell peppers, halved and seeds removed

- 4 oz goat cheese

- 2 tablespoons chopped fresh chives

- 1 tablespoon lemon juice

- Salt and pepper to taste

Prep Time: 15 mins

Cooking Time: 10 mins

Total Time: 25 mins

Servings: 4

Nutrition Facts (per serving):

- Calories: 110

- Fat: 7g

- Saturated fat: 4g

- Cholesterol: 15mg

- Sodium: 130mg

- Carbohydrate: 8g

- Protein: 4g

- Fiber: 2g

Instructions:

1. Preheat oven to 375°F (190°C). Line a baking sheet with parchment paper.

2. In a small bowl, combine goat cheese, chopped fresh chives, lemon juice, salt, and pepper.

3. Stuff each mini bell pepper half with the goat cheese mixture.

4. Place stuffed mini bell peppers on the prepared baking sheet.

5. Bake in the preheated oven for 8-10 minutes, or until the peppers are tender and the cheese is melted and bubbly.

6. Serve stuffed mini bell peppers hot as a delicious and nutritious snack or appetizer option.

Baked Sweet Potato Fries

Ingredients:

- 2 large sweet potatoes, washed and cut into fries

- 1 tablespoon olive oil

- 1 teaspoon garlic powder

- 1 teaspoon paprika

- Salt and pepper to taste

Prep Time: 10 mins

Cooking Time: 25 mins

Total Time: 35 mins

Servings: 4

Nutrition Facts (per serving):

- Calories: 120

- Fat: 3g

- Saturated fat: 0.5g

- Cholesterol: 0mg

- Sodium: 150mg

- Carbohydrate: 22g

- Protein: 2g

- Fiber: 4g

Instructions:

1. Preheat oven to 425°F (220°C). Line a baking sheet with parchment paper.

2. In a large bowl, toss sweet potato fries with olive oil, garlic powder, paprika, salt, and pepper until evenly coated.

3. Arrange seasoned sweet potato fries in a single layer on the prepared baking sheet.

4. Bake in the preheated oven for 20-25 minutes, flipping halfway through, until the fries are golden brown and crispy.

5. Serve baked sweet potato fries hot as a healthier alternative to traditional fries.

Tuna Salad Stuffed Cucumber Cups

Ingredients:

- 2 cucumbers

- 1 can (5 oz) tuna, drained

- 2 tablespoons Greek yogurt

- 1 tablespoon lemon juice

- 1 tablespoon chopped fresh dill

- Salt and pepper to taste

Prep Time: 15 mins

Total Time: 15 mins

Servings: 4

Nutrition Facts (per serving):

- Calories: 90

- Fat: 3g

- Saturated fat: 0.5g

- Cholesterol: 15mg

- Sodium: 200mg

- Carbohydrate: 4g

- Protein: 12g

- Fiber: 1g

Instructions:

1. Cut cucumbers into 2-inch slices and scoop out the seeds to create cups.

2. In a bowl, mix drained tuna, Greek yogurt, lemon juice, chopped fresh dill, salt, and pepper until well combined.

3. Spoon tuna salad into cucumber cups, filling each cup generously.

4. Serve tuna salad stuffed cucumber cups chilled as a light and refreshing snack or appetizer.

Apple and Almond Butter Sandwiches

Ingredients:

- 1 large apple, cored and thinly sliced

- 4 tablespoons almond butter

- 8 whole grain crackers

Prep Time: 5 mins

Total Time: 5 mins

Servings: 2

Nutrition Facts (per serving):

- Calories: 200

- Fat: 12g

- Saturated fat: 1g

- Cholesterol: 0mg

- Sodium: 100mg

- Carbohydrate: 20g

- Protein: 6g

- Fiber: 5g

Instructions:

1. Spread almond butter evenly on 4 whole grain crackers.

2. Top half of the almond butter crackers with thinly sliced apple slices.

3. Place the remaining almond butter crackers on top to form sandwiches.

4. Serve apple and almond butter sandwiches immediately as a delicious and nutritious snack option.

Veggie Sushi Rolls

Ingredients:

- 4 nori seaweed sheets

- 2 cups cooked sushi rice

- 1 small cucumber, julienned

- 1 small carrot, julienned

- 1 avocado, thinly sliced

- Pickled ginger and wasabi for serving (optional)

- Soy sauce for dipping (optional)

Prep Time: 20 mins

Total Time: 20 mins

Servings: 4

Nutrition Facts (per serving):

- Calories: 180

- Fat: 5g

- Saturated fat: 1g

- Cholesterol: 0mg

- Sodium: 200mg

- Carbohydrate: 30g

- Protein: 4g

- Fiber: 4g

Instructions:

1. Place a nori seaweed sheet on a clean surface, shiny side down.

2. Spread a thin layer of cooked sushi rice evenly over the nori sheet, leaving a 1-inch border at the top.

3. Arrange julienned cucumber, carrot, and avocado slices in a line across the bottom third of the rice-covered nori sheet.

4. Roll up the nori sheet tightly, starting from the bottom edge, using a bamboo sushi mat or clean kitchen towel to help shape the roll.

5. Repeat with remaining nori sheets and filling ingredients.

6. Slice each sushi roll into 6-8 pieces using a sharp knife.

7. Serve veggie sushi rolls with pickled ginger, wasabi, and soy sauce for dipping, if desired.

Stuffed Celery Sticks

Ingredients:

- 4 celery stalks, washed and trimmed

- 4 oz cream cheese, softened

- 2 tablespoons chopped fresh chives

- 1 tablespoon lemon juice

- Salt and pepper to taste

- Smoked paprika for garnish

Prep Time: 10 mins

Total Time: 10 mins

Servings: 2

Nutrition Facts (per serving):

- Calories: 100

- Fat: 8g

- Saturated fat: 5g

- Cholesterol: 25mg

- Sodium: 150mg

- Carbohydrate: 4g

- Protein: 2g

- Fiber: 1g

Instructions:

1. In a bowl, mix softened cream cheese, chopped fresh chives, lemon juice, salt, and pepper until smooth and well combined.

2. Spread the cream cheese mixture evenly into the hollowed-out center of each celery stalk.

3. Sprinkle stuffed celery sticks with smoked paprika for added flavor and garnish.

4. Serve stuffed celery sticks chilled as a crunchy and satisfying snack option.

DESSERT AND TREATS RECIPES

Baked Apples with Cinnamon and Walnuts

Ingredients:

- 4 large apples (such as Granny Smith or Honeycrisp)

- 1/4 cup chopped walnuts

- 2 tablespoons honey or maple syrup

- 1 teaspoon ground cinnamon

- 1/4 teaspoon nutmeg

- 1/4 teaspoon vanilla extract

Prep Time: 10 mins

Cooking Time: 25 mins

Total Time: 35 mins

Servings: 4

Nutrition Facts (per serving):

- Calories: 150

- Fat: 3g

- Saturated fat: 0.5g

- Cholesterol: 0mg

- Sodium: 0mg

- Carbohydrate: 32g

- Protein: 1g

- Fiber: 5g

Instructions:

1. Preheat oven to 375°F (190°C). Grease a baking dish with cooking spray.

2. Core the apples and cut a thin slice from the bottom of each apple so they sit flat in the baking dish.

3. In a small bowl, mix chopped walnuts, honey or maple syrup, cinnamon, nutmeg, and vanilla extract.

4. Stuff each apple with the walnut mixture, dividing it evenly among the apples.

5. Place stuffed apples in the prepared baking dish.

6. Bake in the preheated oven for 20-25 minutes, or until apples are tender and fragrant.

7. Serve baked apples with cinnamon and walnuts warm, optionally topped with a dollop of Greek yogurt or a drizzle of honey.

Banana Oatmeal Cookies

Ingredients:

- 2 ripe bananas, mashed

- 1 cup old-fashioned oats

- 1/4 cup chopped nuts (such as walnuts or almonds)

- 2 tablespoons honey or maple syrup

- 1/2 teaspoon ground cinnamon

- 1/4 teaspoon vanilla extract

Prep Time: 10 mins

Cooking Time: 15 mins

Total Time: 25 mins

Servings: 12 cookies

Nutrition Facts (per serving - 1 cookie):

- Calories: 70

- Fat: 2g

- Saturated fat: 0.5g

- Cholesterol: 0mg

- Sodium: 0mg

- Carbohydrate: 13g

- Protein: 2g

- Fiber: 2g

Instructions:

1. Preheat oven to 350°F (175°C). Line a baking sheet with parchment paper.

2. In a mixing bowl, combine mashed bananas, old-fashioned oats, chopped nuts, honey or maple syrup, cinnamon, and vanilla extract.

3. Stir until all ingredients are well combined and form a thick dough.

4. Drop a spoonful of the dough onto the prepared baking sheet, spacing them slightly apart.

5. Flatten each spoonful of dough with the back of a spoon to form cookie shapes.

6. Bake in the preheated oven for 12-15 minutes, or until cookies are golden brown around the edges.

7. Allow banana oatmeal cookies to cool on the baking sheet for 5 minutes before transferring them to a wire rack to cool completely.

Chia Seed Pudding with Mixed Berries

Ingredients:

- 1/4 cup chia seeds

- 1 cup unsweetened almond milk (or any milk of choice)

- 1 tablespoon honey or maple syrup (optional)

- 1/2 teaspoon vanilla extract

- 1 cup mixed berries (such as strawberries, blueberries, raspberries)

Prep Time: 5 mins

Chilling Time: 2 hours

Total Time: 2 hours 5 mins

Servings: 2

Nutrition Facts (per serving):

- Calories: 130

- Fat: 6g

- Saturated fat: 0.5g

- Cholesterol: 0mg

- Sodium: 90mg

- Carbohydrate: 18g

- Protein: 3g

- Fiber: 9g

Instructions:

1. In a mixing bowl, whisk together chia seeds, unsweetened almond milk, honey or maple syrup (if using), and vanilla extract.

2. Let the mixture sit for 5 minutes, then whisk again to prevent clumping.

3. Cover the bowl and refrigerate for at least 2 hours, or until the chia pudding has thickened to a pudding-like consistency.

4. Stir the chia pudding well before serving to redistribute the chia seeds.

5. Divide chia seed pudding into serving cups or bowls and top with mixed berries.

6. Serve chia seed pudding with mixed berries chilled as a healthy and satisfying dessert option.

Greek Yogurt Parfait with Honey and Almonds

Ingredients:

- 1 cup plain Greek yogurt

- 2 tablespoons honey

- 1/4 cup sliced almonds

- 1/4 cup mixed berries (such as strawberries, or blueberries)

Prep Time: 5 mins

Total Time: 5 mins

Servings: 1

Nutrition Facts (per serving):

- Calories: 260

- Fat: 10g

- Saturated fat: 1g

- Cholesterol: 10mg

- Sodium: 60mg

- Carbohydrate: 25g

- Protein: 20g

- Fiber: 3g

Instructions:

1. In a serving glass or bowl, layer plain Greek yogurt, honey, sliced almonds, and mixed berries.

2. Repeat layers until all ingredients are used, ending with a layer of mixed berries on top.

3. Serve Greek yogurt parfait with honey and almonds immediately as a nutritious and delicious dessert or snack option.

Baked Pears with Cinnamon and Walnuts

Ingredients:

- 2 ripe pears, halved and cored

- 1 tablespoon honey or maple syrup

- 1/4 teaspoon ground cinnamon

- 2 tablespoons chopped walnuts

- Greek yogurt or vanilla ice cream for serving (optional)

Prep Time: 10 mins

Cooking Time: 20 mins

Total Time: 30 mins

Servings: 2

Nutrition Facts (per serving):

- Calories: 120

- Fat: 4g

- Saturated fat: 0.5g

- Cholesterol: 0mg

- Sodium: 0mg

- Carbohydrate: 24g

- Protein: 2g

- Fiber: 5g

Instructions:

1. Preheat oven to 375°F (190°C). Place pear halves cut side up in a baking dish.

2. Drizzle honey or maple syrup over the pear halves.

3. Sprinkle ground cinnamon evenly over the pears.

4. Top each pear half with chopped walnuts.

5. Bake in the preheated oven for 15-20 minutes, or until pears are tender and walnuts are lightly toasted.

6. Serve baked pears with cinnamon and walnuts warm, optionally topped with a dollop of Greek yogurt or a scoop of vanilla ice cream.

Chocolate Avocado Mousse

Ingredients:

- 2 ripe avocados

- 1/4 cup unsweetened cocoa powder

- 1/4 cup maple syrup or agave nectar

- 1 teaspoon vanilla extract

- Pinch of salt

- Fresh berries for garnish (optional)

Prep Time: 10 mins

Total Time: 10 mins

Servings: 4

Nutrition Facts (per serving):

- Calories: 200

- Fat: 15g

- Saturated fat: 2g

- Cholesterol: 0mg

- Sodium: 5mg

- Carbohydrate: 19g

- Protein: 3g

- Fiber: 8g

Instructions:

1. Cut the avocados in half, remove the pits, and scoop the flesh into a blender or food processor.

2. Add cocoa powder, maple syrup or agave nectar, vanilla extract, and a pinch of salt to the blender.

3. Blend until smooth and creamy, scraping down the sides as needed.

4. Divide the chocolate avocado mousse into serving cups or bowls.

5. Chill in the refrigerator for at least 30 minutes before serving.

6. Garnish with fresh berries before serving, if desired.

Coconut Chia Seed Pudding

Ingredients:

- 1/4 cup chia seeds

- 1 cup coconut milk

- 1 tablespoon honey or maple syrup

- 1/2 teaspoon vanilla extract

- Shredded coconut for garnish (optional)

- Sliced tropical fruits for topping (such as mango or pineapple)

Prep Time: 5 mins

Chilling Time: 2 hours

Total Time: 2 hours 5 mins

Servings: 2

Nutrition Facts (per serving):

- Calories: 200

- Fat: 15g

- Saturated fat: 10g

- Cholesterol: 0mg

- Sodium: 10mg

- Carbohydrate: 15g

- Protein: 4g

- Fiber: 7g

Instructions:

1. In a mixing bowl, whisk together chia seeds, coconut milk, honey or maple syrup, and vanilla extract.

2. Let the mixture sit for 5 minutes, then whisk again to prevent clumping.

3. Cover the bowl and refrigerate for at least 2 hours, or until the chia pudding has thickened to a pudding-like consistency.

4. Stir the chia pudding well before serving to redistribute the chia seeds.

5. Divide chia seed pudding into serving cups or bowls.

6. Top with shredded coconut and sliced tropical fruits before serving.

Berry Frozen Yogurt Bark

Ingredients:

- 2 cups plain Greek yogurt

- 2 tablespoons honey or maple syrup

- 1 cup mixed berries (such as strawberries, blueberries, raspberries)

- 2 tablespoons unsweetened coconut flakes

Prep Time: 10 mins

Freezing Time: 4 hours

Total Time: 4 hours 10 mins

Servings: 6

Nutrition Facts (per serving):

- Calories: 100

- Fat: 3g

- Saturated fat: 2g

- Cholesterol: 0mg

- Sodium: 20mg

- Carbohydrate: 13g

- Protein: 6g

- Fiber: 2g

Instructions:

1. Line a baking sheet with parchment paper or aluminum foil.

2. In a mixing bowl, stir together Greek yogurt and honey or maple syrup until well combined.

3. Spread the yogurt mixture evenly onto the prepared baking sheet, about 1/4-inch thick.

4. Sprinkle mixed berries and unsweetened coconut flakes over the yogurt mixture.

5. Place the baking sheet in the freezer and freeze for at least 4 hours, or until the yogurt bark is firm.

6. Once frozen, break the yogurt bark into pieces.

7. Serve berry frozen yogurt bark immediately as a refreshing and healthy dessert or snack option.

Almond Flour Banana Bread

Ingredients:

- 2 ripe bananas, mashed

- 2 eggs

- 1/4 cup almond butter

- 1/4 cup honey or maple syrup

- 1 teaspoon vanilla extract

- 1 1/2 cups almond flour

- 1/2 teaspoon baking soda

- 1/2 teaspoon ground cinnamon

- Pinch of salt

Prep Time: 10 mins

Cooking Time: 45 mins

Total Time: 55 mins

Servings: 8

Nutrition Facts (per serving):

- Calories: 220

- Fat: 14g

- Saturated fat: 1.5g

- Cholesterol: 35mg

- Sodium: 120mg

- Carbohydrate: 19g

- Protein: 7g

- Fiber: 3g

Instructions:

1. Preheat oven to 350°F (175°C). Grease a loaf pan with cooking spray or line with parchment paper.

2. In a large mixing bowl, whisk together mashed bananas, eggs, almond butter, honey or maple syrup, and vanilla extract until well combined.

3. In a separate bowl, combine almond flour, baking soda, ground cinnamon, and a pinch of salt.

4. Gradually add the dry ingredients to the wet ingredients, stirring until just combined.

5. Pour the banana bread batter into the prepared loaf pan.

6. Bake in the preheated oven for 40-45 minutes, or until a toothpick inserted into the center comes out clean.

7. Allow almond flour banana bread to cool in the pan for 10 minutes before transferring it to a wire rack to cool completely.

Coconut Mango Rice Pudding

Ingredients:

- 1 cup cooked brown rice

- 1 cup coconut milk

- 1 ripe mango, diced

- 2 tablespoons honey or maple syrup

- 1/2 teaspoon vanilla extract

- Shredded coconut for garnish (optional)

Prep Time: 10 mins

Cooking Time: 20 mins

Total Time: 30 mins

Servings: 2

Nutrition Facts (per serving):

- Calories: 280

- Fat: 10g

- Saturated fat: 9g

- Cholesterol: 0mg

- Sodium: 5mg

- Carbohydrate: 45g

- Protein: 3g

- Fiber: 4g

Instructions:

1. In a saucepan, combine cooked brown rice, coconut milk, diced mango, honey or maple syrup, and vanilla extract.

2. Cook over medium heat, stirring occasionally, until the mixture is heated through and the flavors are well combined, about 10-15 minutes.

3. Remove from heat and let cool slightly.

4. Divide coconut mango rice pudding into serving bowls.

5. Garnish with shredded coconut before serving, if desired.

6. Serve coconut mango rice pudding warm or chilled as a tropical-inspired dessert option.

14-DAY MEAL PLAN

Day 1:

- *Breakfast:* Chia Seed Pudding with Mixed Berries
- *Lunch:* Greek Yogurt Parfait with Honey and Almonds
- *Dinner:* Baked Pears with Cinnamon and Walnuts

Day 2:

- *Breakfast:* Coconut Chia Seed Pudding
- *Lunch:* Berry Frozen Yogurt Bark
- *Dinner:* Almond Flour Banana Bread

Day 3:

- *Breakfast:* Chocolate Avocado Mousse
- *Lunch:* Coconut Mango Rice Pudding
- *Dinner:* Baked Pears with Cinnamon and Walnuts

Day 4:

- *Breakfast:* Banana Oatmeal Cookies
- *Lunch:* Berry Frozen Yogurt Bark
- *Dinner:* Almond Flour Banana Bread

Day 5:

- *Breakfast:* Chocolate Avocado Mousse

- *Lunch:* Greek Yogurt Parfait with Honey and Almonds
- *Dinner:* Coconut Mango Rice Pudding

Day 6:

- *Breakfast:* Baked Apples with Cinnamon and Walnuts
- *Lunch:* Berry Frozen Yogurt Bark
- *Dinner:* Almond Flour Banana Bread

Day 7:

- *Breakfast:* Banana Oatmeal Cookies
- *Lunch:* Coconut Chia Seed Pudding
- *Dinner:* Chocolate Avocado Mousse

Day 8:

- *Breakfast:* Coconut Chia Seed Pudding
- *Lunch:* Greek Yogurt Parfait with Honey and Almonds
- *Dinner:* Baked Pears with Cinnamon and Walnuts

Day 9:

- *Breakfast:* Banana Oatmeal Cookies
- *Lunch:* Berry Frozen Yogurt Bark
- *Dinner:* Almond Flour Banana Bread

Day 10:

- *Breakfast:* Chocolate Avocado Mousse

- *Lunch:* Coconut Mango Rice Pudding

- *Dinner:* Baked Pears with Cinnamon and Walnuts

Day 11:

- *Breakfast:* Chia Seed Pudding with Mixed Berries

- *Lunch:* Berry Frozen Yogurt Bark

- *Dinner:* Almond Flour Banana Bread

Day 12:

- *Breakfast:* Banana Oatmeal Cookies

- *Lunch:* Greek Yogurt Parfait with Honey and Almonds

- *Dinner:* Coconut Mango Rice Pudding

Day 13:

- *Breakfast:* Chocolate Avocado Mousse

- *Lunch:* Berry Frozen Yogurt Bark

- *Dinner:* Almond Flour Banana Bread

Day 14:

- *Breakfast:* Baked Apples with Cinnamon and Walnuts

- *Lunch:* Coconut Chia Seed Pudding

- *Dinner:* Chocolate Avocado Mousse

CONCLUSION

In conclusion, adopting a supercharged diverticulitis diet tailored for seniors can significantly contribute to better health outcomes and improved quality of life. By incorporating a variety of nutrient-rich foods, including whole grains, lean proteins, fruits, vegetables, and healthy fats, seniors can support their digestive health and overall well-being.

Throughout this journey, we've explored the importance of understanding diverticulitis, its causes, symptoms, and available treatment options. We've also delved into the crucial role that diet plays in both the prevention and management of diverticulitis, focusing on foods to include and avoid to maintain digestive health.

Moreover, we've provided practical tips on essential tools and equipment for meal preparation, as well as various cooking methods that promote healthy eating among seniors. By empowering individuals with knowledge and resources, we aim to inspire confidence in navigating dietary choices and fostering a positive relationship with food.

Furthermore, we've curated a collection of delicious and nutritious recipes suitable for every mealtime occasion, ensuring that seniors can enjoy flavourful and satisfying dishes while adhering to their dietary requirements. From breakfast to dessert, each recipe offers a balance of essential nutrients and mouthwatering flavors, making healthy eating an enjoyable and sustainable lifestyle choice.